CAREER AS A

BIOMEDICAL EQUIPMENT TECHNICIAN

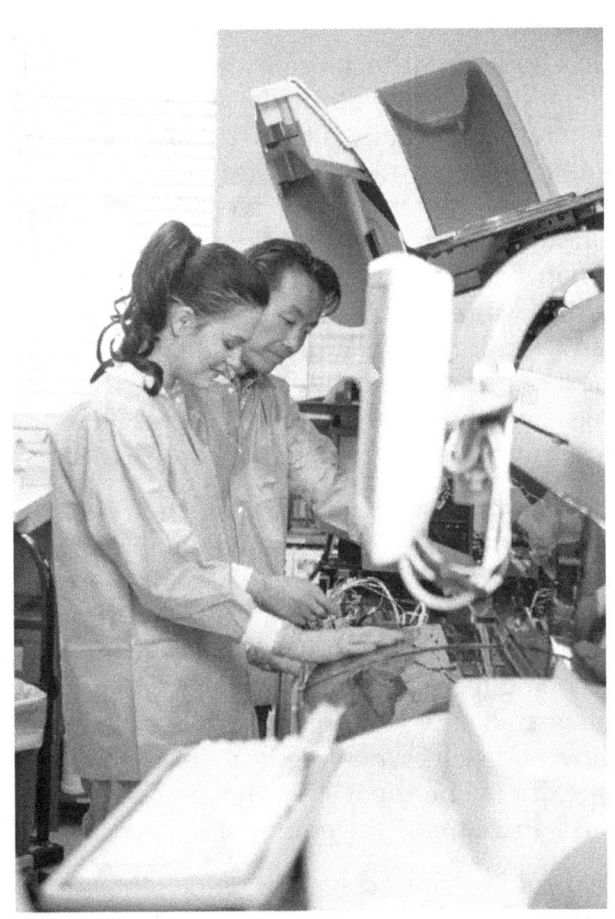

EVERY DAY, COUNTLESS LIVES DEPEND on life-saving medical apparatus. Hospital rooms, surgery suites, and emergency rooms are filled with technological wonders like defibrillators, ventilators, and heart monitors. If any one of these machines breaks down, a person's life could be at risk. Keeping them up and running properly is the responsibility of biomedical equipment technicians. These professionals, also known as BMETS, are highly skilled in the installation and repair of a wide variety of modern medical equipment.

Some biomedical equipment technicians have generalized skills, while others specialize in particular types of equipment. Generalists are trained to install, inspect, test, calibrate, maintain, repair, and sometimes modify all kinds of biomedical equipment. Junior technicians may start by repairing hydraulic chairs and beds, performing routine maintenance like cleaning monitors, or doing simple calibrations. More experienced BMETs are able to troubleshoot and repair more complex equipment, such as electrosurgical units and anesthesia machines. There are also specialists who work solely on apparatus like dialysis machines, ultrasound scanners, or surgical robots.

Biomedical equipment technicians spend much of their time working hands-on with machines and equipment, but they often have other duties. They may perform some administrative duties like maintaining inventories of parts and components, reviewing product manuals, reordering supplies, and keeping records of maintenance and repair jobs. Those who install new equipment may need to train medical staff how to use it. When medical devices are to be used at home, it may be the BMET who instructs the patient in the use and care of the equipment.

Most biomedical equipment technicians work in hospitals or clinics. Others work in laboratories or manufacturers' facilities. Wherever they work, the environment is exceptionally clean and well equipped. The hours are generally steady, but it is common for BMETs to be on call around the clock for one week out of the month. However, because medical equipment is well maintained, after-hours emergency repair calls do not come often.

It is possible to enter this field with only a high school diploma. Newcomers who have done well in math and science classes may be offered on-the-job training to perform simple tasks. However, most employers prefer candidates with an associate degree. Technicians who have graduated from a biomedical equipment technology or engineering program will have the knowledge and skills to work on most types of medical equipment. They are also eligible to become certified. Certification is voluntary, but it increases your chances of employment and advancement. BMETs who intend to specialize in more sophisticated equipment, such as imaging equipment or laboratory equipment, usually need a bachelor's degree.

As long as there are sick patients depending on complex medical machinery, biomedical equipment technicians will be needed. Experts predict a good job outlook for the foreseeable future. In fact, this is one of the fastest growing occupations that can be entered with an associate degree. Technological advances and the ever-growing demand for healthcare services are pushing the field forward. In addition to hospitals and clinics, a growing number of jobs are expected to be offered by companies that develop and manufacture medical equipment, independent medical research laboratories, third-party service firms, and the military.

A career as a biomedical equipment technician is a good choice for individuals with a mechanical aptitude and an interest in working with the latest technology. It is a constantly changing field that continues to advance in complexity. If you enjoy working with your hands, solving problems, and the idea of spending your days in a medical environment, this may be the career for you.

WHAT YOU CAN DO NOW

HIGH SCHOOL IS AN IMPORTANT TIME for future biomedical equipment technicians. Much of what you can learn now will be useful on the job later, such as courses in industrial arts, computer skills, mechanical drawing, and anything related to electronics. The foundation of your curriculum should be rich in math and science. Biology, chemistry, and physics are basics in the medical environment. You will be dealing with numbers and formulas on a daily basis. Classes in algebra, geometry, and trigonometry will prepare you for that. Shop classes that involve electricity and working machinery will teach you to work with your hands, as well as to follow diagrams and printed instructions. English and any other classes that can help you develop your communications skills will help you deal with the many different people you will interact with on the job.

Research college degree programs. Make sure your curriculum includes all the prerequisites for admission. Admission officers like to see well-rounded applicants. Get involved in extracurricular activities and aim for leadership positions. Consider a bachelor's level program. It may offer more opportunities to work with specialized equipment, such as imaging.

Explore the field. Look for opportunities to job shadow and participate in career fairs. If this looks like something you want to pursue, get some experience. Apply for summer internships and part-time jobs at hospitals and any company that handles biomedical equipment. Join a professional association. For example, the Association for the Advancement of Medical Instrumentation (AAMI) has videos and other career information for students on its website.

HISTORY OF THE CAREER

MEDICAL INSTRUMENTS, HOWEVER PRIMITIVE, have been used since the beginning of human history. The accumulation of medical knowledge over the past several thousand years was accompanied by advances in biomedical equipment. However, most of the scientific research leading to the development of today's complex biomedical equipment happened during the last 200 years.

Physicians and medical researchers have always endeavored to manipulate and monitor the workings of the human body with whatever tools were available at the time, but medical equipment and instruments remained crude until the Industrial Revolution. The 18th century saw the discovery of medical instruments that, for the first time, could monitor many subtle processes of the human body with relative precision. As more instruments were developed, medical professionals increasingly demanded more consistency and reliability. By the middle of the 19th century, at the heights of the Industrial Revolution, the modern medical equipment manufacturing industry was well established.

For the next 100 years, medical researchers greatly increased their knowledge of the chemical and electrical nature of the human body. What they learned necessitated progressively more sophisticated equipment.

It was during this time that the clinical engineering field began, with highly trained individuals supplying the manufacturers with new inventions and designs for improved medical equipment. At the same time, those new instruments and equipment needed someone to introduce them, install them, and make sure they continued to work properly. That someone would be a trained biomedical equipment technician.

Training was first provided by the manufacturers, but as more equipment became standardized, it became possible to offer specialized training through schools and vocational training centers. The US Surgeon General authorized one of the first such training programs in 1943, at the height of World War II. The three-month course, conducted at the St. Louis Medical Depot, was the origin of the US Army's Biomedical Training School. It was the first training program in the country to cover a wide variety of medical equipment rather than the few devices a particular manufacturer produced.

Perhaps the single most important decade, so far, for biomedical technology was the 1950s. Right from the start, the growth of the biomedical technology field was remarkable. The focus was on two things: mechanization and automation. Mechanization began in the Industrial Revolution with the production of pumps, motors, bellows, control arms, and other mechanisms needed to construct biomedical equipment. Over the years, mechanisms were improved and perfected, but it was not until the 1950s that automation was applied to the process. It was during this time that medical researchers started to develop new technologies that would help increase productivity and reduce laboratory processing times. There had long been reports of individual scientists creating automated devices for their own use in the laboratory. During the 1950s, medical researchers started developing machines that could automate processes in the hospital environment, such as analyzing blood components or preparing tissue specimens for microscopic examination. By the end of the Second World War, every hospital had multiple types of automated equipment.

Other advances that took hold in the 1950s were in the field of electronics. Until this time, all medical equipment was mechanical. That changed with the invention of the electron microscope in 1950 and the heart-lung machine in 1953. Automated devices would not have progressed very far without electronics. Prior to the 1950s, few hospitals had any electronic medical devices. Today, any good size hospital has thousands.

As medical equipment became more sophisticated, the demand for trained technicians grew. The availability and scope of training programs expanded in the 1960s. In 1962, the first organized in-hospital training program was established at Sinai Hospital in Baltimore. A year later, the US Army BMET School moved to larger headquarters in Denver where it could train more people to work with advanced medical equipment technology. In 1967, the US Office of Education backed the founding of the Technical Education Research Center where a two-year post-high school curriculum for BMETs was developed.

Consumer advocate Ralph Nader is often credited with firmly establishing biomedical equipment technician as a distinct, valued profession. In 1970, Nader wrote an article that was published in *Ladies Home Journal*. He spoke of unsafe hospitals and the thousands of patients killed or injured by undetected electrocutions every year. The article was shocking. It prompted independent research into the danger of "micro-shock," which eventually led to the creation of standards for electrical safety in hospitals. This gave a big push to the hiring of biomedical equipment technicians who would ensure that their employing hospitals were always in compliance.

Evolution of Biomedical Equipment Technology

Biomedical equipment is an ever increasing part of healthcare. In the US alone, more than $150 billion a year is spent on medical devices. Technology continues to push the field forward with more technologically complex machines being put in our hospitals and healthcare centers every year. With each advance, new challenges await the professionals who are responsible for ensuring it works without fail.

The first technicians were skilled assistants who learned a trade and went to work for an engineer or scientist who happened to be somehow involved in the medical equipment industry. The next generation of technicians learned and applied a single technology, such as mechanics. Biomedical equipment technicians are now trained in at least two fields of science and technology, which means, at minimum, electronics and human physiology. Today's biomedical equipment technicians need to be ready to deal with everything from miniaturization borrowed from space technology, to "smart" medical equipment, to robotics. Those who are ready and willing to stay up to date will always be valued members of the healthcare team.

WHERE YOU WILL WORK

THE NUMBER OF EMPLOYED BMETS is quickly approaching 50,000. They usually work in hospitals, medical centers, and large clinics where there is high-tech equipment and instruments. Only about 15 percent are actually employed by the hospitals where they work. Instead they are hired by companies on the supply side, such as biomedical equipment manufacturers, wholesale suppliers, or third-party service firms. Other employers include research institutes, biological laboratories, and health and personal care stores. Government hospitals and the military also employ biomedical equipment technicians. Approximately 15 percent of technicians are self-employed.

BMETs employed by hospitals or large medical centers work in the biomedical or clinical engineering department. Those working for manufacturers or wholesalers might be in the sales, service, or engineering department.

Most BMETs work here in the states, but there are opportunities to work elsewhere in the world. The best places are third world countries where trained BMETs are rare, but where hospitals are being outfitted with biomedical equipment. All equipment breaks down at some point, so anyone willing to spend time in such a country can make a good living working for the manufacturer.

Working Conditions

Working conditions for BMETs vary somewhat depending on the employer and type of work being done. Generally, they work in modern, clean medical facilities that are well equipped. They usually have a dedicated workspace with a specially designed workbench and a storage area where tools, commonly used parts, and diagnostic equipment are kept. In the hospital setting, there may be direct contact with patients if the malfunctioning equipment is in use. This exposes technicians to possible risk from communicable diseases, though hospitals have procedures in place to mitigate the risk.

Most BMETs working for hospitals spend all of their time

working at a specific facility. Those who work for equipment manufacturers or equipment maintenance organizations may have to travel a lot between multiple facilities.

Schedules

Most BMETs work full time, 40 hours a week. This may not mean 9-to-5, however. Life-saving medical equipment needs constant monitoring, and any problems need to be fixed immediately. Hospital employees often work outside normal business hours, taking evening, overnight, and weekend shifts. Those who work for equipment suppliers are the most likely to work regular business hours, but even they might be on call some nights and weekends in case emergency repairs are needed.

THE WORK YOU WILL DO

BIOMEDICAL EQUIPMENT IS AN ESSENTIAL PART of today's healthcare. All doctors, either directly or indirectly, rely on various medical devices to run tests, diagnose health issues, and treat patients. Specialty practitioners in particular routinely use increasingly complex equipment that must perform as expected without fail. Biomedical equipment technicians represent an important link between biomedical technology and the healthcare practitioners who depend on it. They are an essential part of the medical team that helps patients recover from medical problems. In extreme circumstances, such as a life support system failure, they can even be life savers.

BMETs install, calibrate, maintain, repair, replace, and operate biomedical equipment. They work with biomedical engineers, medical researchers, physicians, and other healthcare providers.

There are literally thousands of different kinds of biomedical devices. Some are simple, such as electric hospital beds and wheelchairs, but most are more complex. BMETs are trained to work with the newest technology found in laboratories, hospitals, surgery suites, and doctors' offices. They also work with sophisticated dental, optometric, and ophthalmic equipment. Some of the most common devices seen every day by BMETs include patient monitors, kidney machines, vacuum autoclaves (sterilizers), X-ray machines, blood pressure transducers, blood-gas analyzers, pacemakers, defibrillators, and a full range of imaging equipment. In advanced hospitals, they may work on robotic radiosurgery units, CyberKnives, biometric registration cameras, 3-D brain scanners, shockwave lithotripters (used to blast apart kidney stones), and various touchless technologies.

The most advanced equipment is attended to by biomedical equipment technicians who specialize in one kind of equipment. For them, the tools used are very specific to their specialty. However, most BMETs work on a wide variety of medical devices. They might work on a malfunctioning blood-gas analyzer one day and rebuild a dialyzer (artificial kidney) the next.

Much of today's biomedical equipment involves electronics, and that is where most BMETs focus their attention while training for the field. There are also some who are trained in specialty materials, such as plastics for developing artificial organs or blown glass used to craft precision parts for specialized devices.

The job responsibilities of a BMET can be far reaching and varied. The work is generally divided into three phases: installation, maintenance and repairs. Depending on the employer, BMETs might handle all three, but usually they are responsible for one or two.

Installation

BMETs working for biomedical equipment manufacturers install new devices and machines in laboratories and hospitals. In some cases, they review recent installations done by others to make sure they were done correctly. In other cases, they are responsible for handling the entire installation process themselves. Installation procedures follow a basic pattern of setup, testing, calibration, monitoring, and adjustment.

Installation starts with a purchase order. If the particular equipment is new to the BMET, the first step is to review technical manuals and manufacturer's diagrams, and attend training sessions. The new equipment is inspected and tested before it is setup to ensure it complies with performance and safety standards. All biomedical equipment technicians are thoroughly familiar with relevant codes and regulations. Once the equipment is in place, it must be calibrated according to manufacturer's specifications.

After the initial installation, BMETs continue to monitor performance. They may study machine-patient interactions, consult with the healthcare professionals using the equipment, and keep track of manufacturer updates on use. Based on their evaluations, they may determine that modifications are necessary to improve the overall performance of the equipment. Under the direction of medical personnel, it may be necessary to add or change components in order to meet the specific requirements for therapy or diagnosis.

Sometimes BMETs are asked to demonstrate the operation and care of new equipment. Depending on how many people will be using the devices, the instruction may be one-on-one or provided through group Q&A sessions.

Maintenance

Once medical equipment is in place, it must be maintained in good working order. This is a major area of responsibility for biomedical equipment technicians. The goal of BMETs doing this type of work is to prevent problems before they occur and become serious threats to a patient's care. To that end, they conduct routine maintenance. In the hospital setting, that may mean visits to patient rooms, laboratories, operating rooms, and emergencies rooms.

Maintenance can be as simple as checking for worn wires or cleaning the dust out of patient monitoring equipment. It can also be as complicated as troubleshooting a circuit board. The most common maintenance tasks involve vital sign monitors, computer monitors, and defibrillators. During routine maintenance, they may disassemble devices, inspect the components, and reassemble them. They test circuits, clean and lubricate moving parts, and replace worn parts. They recalibrate diagnostic equipment to ensure the accuracy during critical medical tests.

Repairs

The most important work a biomedical equipment technician does is repairing broken machines and faulty instruments. Breakdowns can occur anywhere – hospitals, laboratories, dental offices, or anywhere else medical equipment is found. When a repair order comes in, the BMET springs into action and heads to the location of the offending device. It may be a dental chair that will not recline, a cardiac monitor on the fritz, a leaking anesthesia machine, a blood-gas analyzer giving faulty readings, or any of a thousand other problems. It is the BMET's job to troubleshoot and then repair whatever has gone wrong. Although some technicians are able to fix a variety of equipment, others specialize in repairing one or a small number of specific machines.

The size and scope of a malfunction can vary significantly. Repair orders are prioritized as they come in. Emergency work is placed at the top of the list for immediate attention. Simple calibration or cleaning tasks that may only take an hour or so, are addressed during slower times. Still, the technician will not know for sure the nature of the problem until it is investigated.

The BMET first needs to determine the extent of the malfunction. Troubleshooting is performed using standard and specialized test instruments, such as oscilloscopes, multimeters, and pressure gauges. Sometimes the equipment needs to be disassembled in order to locate the malfunctioning parts.

Most minor malfunctions can be handled immediately. In a hospital setting, there may be a maintenance technician with many replacement parts and components on hand for common repairs. Calibrations are investigated and repaired using specialized test equipment software, something every BMET uses routinely. Major breakdowns may require waiting for replacement parts from the factory. It is the BMET's job to send a written analysis of the problem to the factory and request expedited delivery of needed components.

Most BMETs use ordinary hand tools to make repairs, such as wrenches, screwdrivers, and soldering irons. Computers are used to work on electronic and digital devices. BMETs also refer to factory manuals throughout the repair process. Replacement parts are installed, calibrated, and safety tested according to manufacturers' specifications. When repairs are completed, BMETs are responsible for keeping a record of the repair procedure. In some cases, they may determine it is necessary to notify the manufacturer about possible defects that should be corrected at the factory level.

Those who do repair work are usually the only BMETs who come in contact with patients. This only happens in a hospital setting, when the malfunctioning equipment is in use. Sometimes the technician will invite the input of the patient to help identify the problem. In every case, BMETs must be careful not to disturb patients while going about their job.

Biomedical equipment technicians are also responsible for a variety of other duties. Some manage inventories of all instruments in their facilities, tracking where they are located, who is using them, and their condition after each inspection. They may reorder parts, obtain emergency instruments when needed, and routinely check for safety regulation compliance.

BMETs also work closely with a number of different people. They have discussions with medical staff about equipment problems and the possible need for modifications. They help hospital administrators determine when equipment should be replaced or when new equipment would be worth the investment. They help researchers conduct experiments and collaborate with engineers developing new devices.

Some BMETs choose to get involved in the sales of biomedical equipment. Manufacturers and wholesale suppliers prefer hiring experienced technicians for sales positions because they are deeply familiar with the equipment they would be selling. A sales professional might be better at presenting and closing the deal, but in the medical arena, understanding exactly how the newest equipment can benefit patient care is far more important. The job is simple enough for any good BMET to handle, doing demonstrations and answering questions. BMETs generally get into sales because the potential earnings, which are based primarily on commissions, are greater than a technician's salary.

Specialists

Biomedical equipment technicians are exposed to thousands of different kinds of equipment. Some BMETs are generalists who work with a multitude of machines and instruments, while others specialize in a narrower area such as imaging or laboratory devices. Sometimes this specialization is directed by the employer. For example, it is common for hospitals to assign technicians to a particular department, such as pediatrics, surgery, or renal medicine. Out of necessity, these BMETs become specialists in the particular types of equipment within the department. A technician working in renal medicine, for example, would naturally become an expert on maintaining and repairing dialysis machines.

Other BMETs choose a specialty that interests them, such as robotic surgery, nuclear medicine, artificial organs and prosthetics, telemedicine (including virtual surgery), or healthcare technology management. This usually occurs after working in the field for a while and deciding to get additional training and certification in a specialty area.

The most common specialty is working with imaging equipment. This includes radiographic and fluoroscopic x-ray, LASERs, diagnostic ultrasound, mammography, film image processing, Gamma cameras, positron emission tomography (PET), computed tomography (CT), picture archiving and communication systems (PACS), magnetic resonance imaging (MRI scanning), and nuclear imaging.

Another popular specialty area is maintenance of pulmonary function machines. These include small devices like peak flow monitors and spirometers (instruments that measure air capacity in the lungs), to large complicated machines like PFTs that are the size of small closets. They are used in a variety of environments, including clinics, hospital laboratories, thoracic and cardiopulmonary departments, and rehabilitation centers.

There are also biomedical electronics technicians who specialize in small personal devices designed for patient use, such as blood pressure monitoring systems, sleep apnea machines, and external pacemakers. BMETs working with these devices often make house calls to homebound patients. They regularly check to make sure the devices are working properly and carry replacements with them in case the one in use needs to be fixed. They also instruct patients and their caregivers about correct usage and maintenance.

STORIES OF BMETs ON THE JOB

I Repair Patient Related Equipment in a Hospital

"I work in the medical engineering department. I work on a lot of different kinds of equipment, but the most common are vital signs and telemetry monitors, infusion devices, ventilators, and dialysis machines. Most repairs require nothing more than a screwdriver and Volt Ohm Meter. But I also dig into the electronics, troubleshooting circuit boards and replacing components. Most of what I know about electronics, I learned while interning with a clinical engineer. It's fascinating stuff and I enjoy updating my knowledge with each new advance in the technology.

This is a fast-paced job. I move around the hospital, following through on repair orders as they come in.

There are three other technicians in my department and we are all kept busy throughout the day, every day. When I go to work in the morning, I never know what the day will bring. I like that. It's never boring and always a challenge. It makes the day whiz by. Sometimes a breakdown happens when a patient is in a critical status. In that case, I have to jump on it and get it fixed stat – that means immediately. That can be stressful, but it's also very satisfying to be able to take care of it. In a small way, I think of myself as a hero.

A lot of wannabe technicians just want to work with tools and machines. There are some BMET jobs like that, but the hospital environment is different. I work closely with people all day long. I enjoy working with the nurses and occasionally chatting with the patients. You have to be a people person here, and I am.

This is a great job, with good pay and super benefits. My advice to anyone thinking about getting into this field is to jump in sooner rather than later. The need is great and jobs are pretty easy to find. You don't even have to wait until you have a college degree. You can start an internship straight out of high school, but only if you can demonstrate some mechanical aptitude. You do need to make the most of high school. There is a lot of math and science involved in this work so concentrate on those kinds of classes. And do enroll in a training program at your local community college or vocational school as soon as you feel ready. You will need that degree down the road to get certified and pursue advancement. Without it, you will be stuck in a low-level job until you do."

I Am a Traveling BMET

"A lot of BMETs have to travel. Most just go from facility to facility, installing new equipment or doing routine maintenance. I chose to venture a little farther out. I work for a manufacturer that sends me to countries all over the world, to service their medical equipment wherever it may be. I've been to some interesting cities in Europe, but mostly I am needed in third world countries.

Most biomedical equipment is manufactured in the US, Japan, and Europe, but it is installed everywhere there are hospitals or clinics. Modern biomedical equipment is designed to be used in clean, air-conditioned environments with reliable electricity. Even in the best facilities in the most advanced countries, equipment needs regular maintenance and skilled technicians to make repairs. Medical facilities in third world countries have to deal with intense heat, dust, power surges and outages, and humidity. The problem is there are no training programs for BMETs in these places. That's why I am needed.

I never know what I'm going to run into on a new assignment. The problems are often more basic than here in the states. In Africa, for example, I was sent to repair an X-ray machine that wasn't working. Within a couple of minutes, I discovered a faulty power supply. Sometimes I'm sent to check on recently installed equipment only to discover it has never been used because nobody there knew how. They couldn't read or couldn't understand the user manual.

The conditions I work in are less than ideal – lack of supplies and parts, limited access to tools (must bring your own!), questionable sanitation, language issues, and sketchy electrical circuits. I could be in a comfortable, modern hospital, never breaking a sweat, but the rewards of my overseas work can't be measured. It is my privilege to play such a critical role in the developing world hospitals. I know for a fact that my work saves lives."

PERSONAL QUALIFICATIONS

THE MEDICAL EQUIPMENT INDUSTRY grows bigger every year, and so does the need for more biomedical equipment technicians to keep the machines up and running. It is a tremendous opportunity for the right type of person, but the work is not for everyone. It takes a unique mix of technological skills and soft skills. Here are some personality traits that most often describe successful BMETs.

Technophiles

A keen interest in technology, especially anything new, is a basic necessity in this field. BMETs are typically the people who figured out computers long before high school and gleefully disassembled (and reassembled) every gadget they got their hands on. Medical equipment is often very complex, integrating precise machinery and advanced computer programs. That means BMETs have to apply both mechanical skills and software proficiency to keep machines up and running. They often use sophisticated diagnostic tools to troubleshoot problems, and then dive into the nuts and bolts to get the job done.

People Person

The word "technician" is associated with mechanical work, but good biomedical technicians are usually working in a hospital environment where strong people skills come in handy. They often do their work in the presence of a patient and just like doctors, a good bedside manner is appreciated. Some days can be rough, especially when complicated emergency repairs are called for. The doctors and nurses may be stressed because a life-saving machine is not working properly. The patient may be scared and lash out. In these situations, a dose of compassion is called for. Experienced BMETs always keep the human factor in mind, knowing that what they do will make everyone feel better.

Good Communicators

A BMET's job is not performed in a vacuum. There is a great deal of interaction with manufacturers, medical professionals, hospital staff, administrators, supervisors, coworkers, and patients. Effective communications skills are vital when imparting technical information, whether by phone, in writing, or in person. Some people will understand technical jargon, but others will not. The BMET needs to know how to break it down to layman's language. A significant amount of time is spent meeting with hospital administrators and training medical personnel to use equipment. When equipment needs extensive repairs or is in need of replacement, the BMET must be able to describe the situation quickly and clearly to the administrator and/or the manufacturer.

Problem Solvers

Most of the time, BMETs do installations and routine maintenance, but when something goes wrong, they are called in to troubleshoot the problem and fix it. They have technical skills and diagnostic tools to identify most problems easily. As medical equipment becomes more complex, problems become more difficult to identify. Good BMETs see every problem as a puzzle. They solve puzzles with creative thinking and making sure that no detail goes unnoticed.

Reliable

In the medical world, time is of the essence. People depend on BMETs to be on time, every time they are called in. Reliability is especially important for those who do repair work. Because the need to get vital medical equipment up and running again is urgent, being late can literally mean the difference between life and death. Good BMETs are able to work quickly, even in high-pressure situations.

ATTRACTIVE FEATURES

OVERALL, BMETS REPORT THAT THEY are very satisfied with their career choice. They have good reasons for being happy – good pay for minimal training, excellent benefits, and job security. Many enter the field for these reasons, but experienced BMETs cite additional sources of job satisfaction.

One of the biggest benefits of being a biomedical technician is being able to help people in a very significant way. The work BMETs do often impacts the outcome of patient care. These professionals are responsible for ensuring the proper function of life support systems such as heart-lung machines, defibrillators, heart monitors, intravenous (IV) machines, and imaging equipment like ultrasound and MRI scanners. These devices are essential for administering quality care that could make the difference between life and death.

BMETs are acutely aware of this, especially when attending to equipment that is in use. In that situation, they often interact directly with patients and see first-hand the reason their work is so valuable.

BMETs get to work with the newest, cutting edge technology. Hospitals strive to offer the most innovative technology available, partly because the public demands it and because healthcare is a competitive environment. The type of person who becomes a successful biomedical equipment technician finds the introduction of new equipment exciting. They are eager to learn and master new technologies and do so through on-the-job training, seminars, manufacturer training classes, and self-study.

This is an easy entry career that does not require a college education. That does not mean BMETs are stuck in low-level, mundane jobs. There are many opportunities for advancement. With just a few years of experience, a BMET can get promoted into a supervisory role. From there, management positions may be offered. At any time, a BMET can stand out by getting certification in a specialty area. Such certification opens up more job opportunities and provides higher pay.

UNATTRACTIVE ASPECTS

TECHNICALLY MINDED PEOPLE WHO WOULD prefer working with machines rather than interacting with people may not be suited for this job. Most BMETs work in a hospital setting, where they often need to work around patients when equipment is in use. Those who are not great communicators would probably find that an uncomfortable situation. In addition to patients, they also have to interact with numerous other healthcare personnel, supervisors, and manufacturers.

This job does not necessarily end at 5:00. Medical equipment is used around the clock and can malfunction at any time. Technicians are often on call after hours to handle emergency repairs. Others are scheduled for night and weekend shifts, usually on a rotating basis.

The work can be stressful. Medical environments get intense when vital medical equipment is down. When a heart-monitoring machine quits functioning, for example, a patient's life depends on the machine being repaired immediately. There is no room for error and no time to spare. The BMET has to quickly apply problem-solving skills while working under pressure – sometimes while the patient is still attached to the machine.

The biomedical equipment industry is becoming more diverse. The most successful BMETs are trained to work with a wide variety of equipment. It usually takes a couple of years in a community college or vocational school to get this kind of training. Sometimes the training a technician receives is specific to the equipment from a particular manufacturer or used in one type of workplace. This usually happens to someone who enters the field straight out of high school. The knowledge they receive may be in-depth, making them experts on that type of equipment. That can be limiting when looking for a new job. In this situation, technicians can be stuck in place until they get more training, which usually means going back to school.

EDUCATION AND TRAINING

EDUCATION REQUIREMENTS FOR BIOMEDICAL equipment technicians vary, depending on the type of work that will be done. Simpler tasks may only require a high school diploma and some on-the-job training. However, to go beyond repairing hospital beds and electric wheelchairs, an associate degree in biomedical equipment technology or engineering is needed. Advancing to more complex equipment, such as MRI scanners and defibrillators, usually requires a bachelor's degree.

Graduate degrees are also needed in certain circumstances. For example, if a four-year college graduate wants to conduct research or design new biomedical equipment, a master's degree in clinical engineering may be required. Those who want to get into the business side and advance into general management may want to pursue an MBA (Master of Business Administration).

Most biomedical equipment technicians start with a two-year associate degree in biomedical equipment technology or engineering. To be eligible for eventual certification, aspiring technicians should choose a BMET degree program that is accredited by ABET (Accreditation Board for Engineering and Technology) or the ATMAE (Association of Technology, Management, and Applied Engineering). Students in these programs are trained on a series of biomedical devices, each more complex than the last. Each piece of equipment is different, and must be learned separately. This usually means studying the manufacturer's technical specifications and operating manual.

Extensive hands-on instruction is the hallmark of BMET training. Accredited programs are offered by vocational schools and community colleges that have partnered with local hospitals where students can get experience working on sensitive biomedical equipment in the field. Internships are strongly advised and can be arranged through the school.

Once on the job, new graduates observe and assist experienced BMETs for several months. As they learn and master certain tasks, they become more independent, but may still work under supervision for up to a year.

BMETs should plan on continuing their education as they are responsible for staying current with changes in their field. Biomedical equipment technology is always evolving and new devices are introduced often. To keep up with new technologies, BMETs study equipment manuals and attend seminars offered by biomedical device manufacturers. In some cases, employers and manufacturers provide on-the-job training for new equipment.

Military Training

In addition to vocational schools and community colleges, the military is an excellent source of training in biomedical equipment technology. Comprehensive BMET training is available to all members of the three branches of the armed forces. The military's BMET training is conducted at Fort Sam Houston and is a part of the Military Education and Training Campus (METC). It is a rigorous program that lasts for 10 months. Upon completion, trainees return to their individual services (Army, Navy, or Air Force).

Certifications

Although not mandatory, certification is strongly encouraged. Most employers prefer candidates who are certified because it demonstrates they possess the knowledge and skills needed to perform the work.

Certification also increases a working BMET's chances for advancement. There is no reason not to pursue it since most manufacturers and employers, especially hospitals, will cover any costs associated with certification.

Most BMETs obtain their certification through the Association for the Advancement of Medical Instrumentation (AAMI). The basic certification for generalists is the Certified Biomedical Equipment Technician (CBET). A CBET is recognized in the technical community as proof of competence across many facets of the field. Candidates for this certification must have an associate degree in biomedical equipment technology from an accredited program and pass an examination from the International Certification Commission (ICC).

There are also certifications offered by other professional associations, including the Certified Biomedical Auditor (CBA) from the American Society of Quality or a Biomedical Electronics Technician certification (CBET) from the Electronics Technician Association (ETA).

Specialized Certification

Some BMETs choose to specialize in certain types of biomedical technology. To advance into these areas, specialized certification is needed. There are four specialty certifications available:

Certified Radiology Equipment Specialist (CRES) in diagnostic imaging, nuclear medicine equipment or radiological equipment

Certified Laboratory Equipment Specialists (CLES) for work that involves the many different kinds of equipment found in medical laboratory environments

Certified Nephrology Equipment Specialist (CNES) that covers equipment used in nephrology, such as hemodialysis machines

Certified Healthcare Technology Manager (CHTM) for those in management of healthcare technology operations as well as the management of personnel

To earn any of these credentials, candidates must meet educational requirements, pass a computer-based examination, and fulfill specific work experience requirements.

EARNINGS

BMETS HAVE SEEN THEIR SALARIES RISE year after year. While the average annual income for all BMETs is around $60,000, actual wages range from the low $30,000s to a high of almost $90,000. Most of the difference lies in the level of training and experience.

Entry-level pay is around $20 an hour on average, but may range from $15 to $25 depending on location. On a yearly basis, that works out to $32,000 to $58,000. Mid-level BMETS average $54,000, and senior professionals earn about $66,000 nationwide. Those earning more than $80,000 are typically managers or those certified to work with imaging equipment.

Those in supervisory or senior positions are at the top of the salary scale. To push earnings even higher, experienced BMETs can expect a significant raise in pay by advancing to a Biomedical Engineering Manager position. This usually means going back to school for more training, but the investment of time and money is worth it. The pay can be as much as twice that of the average BMET!

Aside from training and experience, the single biggest factor that determines how much a BMET can expect to be paid is the type of employer. The median yearly wages paid in the top five industries that employ BMETs are as follows:

- Hospitals, both public and private
  $68,000

- Medical equipment wholesale suppliers
  $50,000

- Electronics and precision equipment repair and maintenance firms
  $40,000

- Outpatient healthcare services
  $46,000

- Health and personal care retailers
  $36,000

The industry that pays the most is medical device manufacturing, where BMETs routinely earn more than $85,000. However, this industry has the smallest number of jobs to offer and the competition is intense.

The size of the employer also makes a difference. For example, hospitals with more than 15 BMETS on staff pay up to $15,000 a year more than those with fewer than five.

One way BMETs boost overall income is through overtime pay, which is time-and-a-half for any hours beyond 40 in a given week. Anyone who wants to earn some extra money this way can easily do so. Although BMETs work regular daytime hours most of the time, they are often expected to be on call during the off hours. Equipment can break down anytime of the day or night, or on weekends. It may be an inconvenience, but BMETs are paid well for coming in during their down time and taking care of the problem.

Nearly all BMETs receive good benefits, with most packages including health, dental, vision, and life insurance. Most employers also offer tuition reimbursement – a good thing to know since more training could mean more pay. Profit sharing is also common among those who work for manufacturers and suppliers (not hospitals that are usually nonprofit).

There may be bonuses and commissions, particularly for those involved in sales. Annual year-end bonuses can average $2,000. Commissions vary a lot, but generally exceed $2,000 a year.

OPPORTUNITIES

GROWTH IN THE BIOMEDICAL TECHNOLOGY FIELD is expected to continue for the foreseeable future. In fact, it is one of the fastest growing occupations that can be entered with only an associate degree. The increasing number of job openings is a result of technological advances and the public's demand for healthcare services. As long as there are hospitals and sick patients, there will be jobs for skilled biomedical equipment technicians. Hospitals, service maintenance organizations, and equipment manufacturers will offer most job openings for new graduates.

The aging population in the US has been growing steadily over the past decade as baby boomers started reaching 60. As people age, they generally need more medical care. Millions of baby boomers and other older adults have created significant pressure on the healthcare system, demanding whatever it takes to remain active and live longer. The health professionals who take care of them are prescribing more complex tests and are performing more advanced procedures that require complicated equipment.

Changes in technology have resulted in many new kinds of medical equipment. Biomedical equipment is no longer solely found in large hospitals either. There are sophisticated devices utilizing computer technology in dental offices, optometry offices, and family practice clinics. At the same time, the biomedical equipment found in hospitals is increasingly more difficult to maintain. Although there will always be a place for technicians to work on simpler equipment like electric hospital beds, the outlook is especially favorable for BMETs with a thorough knowledge of software and electronics. The highest demand and the highest pay are for those who are trained and certified to work on imaging equipment, such as electrocardiograms and ultrasounds.

Biomedical technology jobs are everywhere, but opportunities are greatest for those who are willing to relocate. Hospitals and clinics in small towns and rural areas, for example, typically see few qualified applicants. There are also opportunities for those who want to see the world. Biomedical equipment is everywhere, even third world countries. Many locations desperately need trained BMETs to service that equipment when it inevitably fails. More and more of the manufacturers who provide that equipment are hiring BMETs to fill the gap. There is little, if any, difference between biomedical equipment used here in the US and in other countries. A malfunctioning MRI scanner in Texas will be diagnosed and fixed the same way as one in an undeveloped African nation. A trained BMET can literally work anywhere.

Opportunities for advancement are plentiful. At some point, BMETs outgrow the need for supervision and may eventually be promoted to supervisory positions themselves. In some cases, particularly if they have expertise in a specialty area, they may become instructors, assist in research, or take on managerial responsibilities. Some positions may require additional education and certification. Employers will often cover the associated costs.

Experienced BMETs sometimes pursue more opportunities through self-employment. That may mean starting a business with a staff of junior technicians to do the work, or it could simply mean venturing out on your own as a freelancer doing work for multiple facilities.

GETTING STARTED

IT IS NEVER TOO EARLY TO START THE PROCESS of finding your first job as a BMET. Begin by making as many networking contacts as you can. Your first contacts will be your teachers. Most instructors will either be active in the field or have an extensive background as a working professional. Either way, they can point you in the right direction to start your job search.

Valuable contacts can also be made through internships and volunteer positions. Some colleges require an internship to qualify for graduation. In that case, they usually provide assistance in finding an internship program. You can also locate your own internship through hospitals, medical equipment manufacturers, and third party service firms. For volunteer opportunities, go to the nearest hospital. The biggest volunteer organizations offering opportunities in technical service departments are found through hospitals. If the volunteer organization does not list any appropriate positions, go directly to the department heads and offer your services. In addition to networking opportunities, interning and volunteering provide experience in a relevant work environment and exposure to details such as medical jargon that will impress potential future employers. In some cases, interns may be hired for full-time positions.

Join professional associations such as the Advancement of Medical Instrumentation (AAMI) and Medical Equipment and Technology Association (META). Not only do these organizations offer plenty of networking opportunities, but they also post open positions on their websites. Do not overlook local and regional associations. For example, California residents should consider joining the California Medical Instrumentation Association (CMIA), which maintains a list of open positions.

Check with your school's career resource center. There you will find job postings and notices of upcoming job fairs. You can also get help with writing résumés and pick up some interview tips.

Apply directly to hospitals, manufacturers, and third party maintenance firms. For hospitals, contact the department head for biomed departments. The ones you want are usually called Biomedical or Clinical Engineering. Some hospitals maintain searchable databases of open positions, while others hire only through a designated agency. Every OEM (Original Equipment Manufacturer) in the biomed industry maintains a staff of Field Service Technicians (FST) to install, upgrade, and maintain their equipment. Most OEMs have websites with portals to the company hiring process. Third party maintenance organizations operate within the hospital environment, either replacing the hospital's entire onsite biomedical or clinical engineering department, or maintaining only the equipment installed by certain manufacturers. These organizations are a tremendous resource for new BMETs – the larger ones employ hundreds of new graduates. Contact the managers of local branches. If there are no immediate openings, ask for consideration when something does develop.

ASSOCIATIONS

■ **Accreditation Board for Engineering and Technology (ABET)**
http://www.abet.org

■ **American Society of Quality**
www.asq.org

■ **Association for the Advancement of Medical Instrumentation**
http://www.aami.org/student

■ **Association of Technology, Management, and Applied Engineering (ATMAE)**
http://www.atmae.org

■ **Electronics Technician Association (ETA)**
http://www.eta-i.org

■ **Medical Equipment & Technology Association (META)**
http://www.mymeta.org

PERIODICAL

■ **24x7 Magazine**
http://www.24x7mag.com

WEBSITE

■ **TriMedx Foundation**
http://www.trimedxfoundation.org

www.ingramcontent.com/pod-product-compliance
Lightning Source LLC
Chambersburg PA
CBHW070522220526
45467CB00002B/792